GLUTEN

FREE FOOD

LIST

TABLE OF CONTENT

A gluten-free diet involves avoiding gluten, a protein found in wheat, barley, rye, and their derivatives. This dietary approach isn't just a trend; it's crucial for individuals with celiac disease, a severe autoimmune disorder triggered by gluten consumption. When those with celiac disease eat gluten, their immune system responds by damaging the small intestine's lining, leading to malabsorption of nutrients and various health issues.

However, it's not limited to celiac disease alone. Non-celiac gluten sensitivity affects individuals who experience symptoms similar to those with celiac disease but lack the same immune response. For them, eliminating gluten from their diet alleviates digestive problems, fatigue, and other discomforts.

Transitioning to a gluten-free lifestyle involves more than simply avoiding bread and pasta. It requires a keen understanding of food labels, as gluten hides in unexpected products like sauces, dressings, and even certain medications. Luckily, an increasing awareness of gluten-related disorders has led to a surge in available gluten-free alternatives, from grains like quinoa and rice to

dedicated gluten-free versions of traditionally
gluten-containing foods.

Embracing a gluten-free diet involves not just
substituting gluten-containing foods but also
ensuring a balanced and varied intake to meet
nutritional needs. With the right information and
resources, navigating a gluten-free lifestyle can
lead to improved health and well-being for those
sensitive or intolerant to gluten.

DEFINITION OF GLUTEN FREE

A gluten-free diet involves the complete avoidance
of gluten. For a product to be labeled gluten-free, it
must contain less than 20 parts per million (ppm)
of gluten, as recognized by regulatory standards in
many countries.

Gluten serves as a binding agent, providing
elasticity to dough and contributing to the chewy
texture of many baked goods. However, for
individuals with celiac disease or gluten sensitivity,
consuming even trace amounts of gluten can
trigger adverse reactions, leading to intestinal
damage, inflammation, and a range of symptoms
like abdominal pain, bloating, fatigue, and skin
issues.

Gluten-free foods encompass a broad spectrum, including naturally gluten-free items like fruits, vegetables, legumes, and unprocessed meats, as well as specially manufactured gluten-free versions of traditional products like bread, pasta, and snacks. The latter often rely on alternative flours like rice, almond, or tapioca to replicate the texture and taste of gluten-containing counterparts.

The growing prevalence of gluten-related disorders has prompted increased awareness and availability of gluten-free options in grocery stores, restaurants, and food establishments. While adhering to a gluten-free diet can pose challenges in terms of label reading and meal planning, it's become more manageable with the expansion of gluten-free offerings and greater public understanding of these dietary needs.

ADVANTAGES

Adopting a gluten-free lifestyle can offer several advantages, particularly for those with celiac disease or gluten sensitivity. First and foremost, eliminating gluten can alleviate uncomfortable and sometimes debilitating symptoms such as gastrointestinal issues, fatigue, joint pain, and skin problems. It aids in promoting digestive health by reducing inflammation in the gut.

A gluten-free diet often encourages individuals to consume more whole and unprocessed foods like fruits, vegetables, lean proteins, and gluten-free grains, potentially leading to a healthier overall diet. Many individuals report increased energy levels and improved concentration after eliminating gluten from their meals, contributing to a better quality of life.

The rising awareness of gluten-related disorders has spurred the food industry to develop a wider range of gluten-free products, making it easier for those with specific dietary needs to find suitable and flavorful alternatives. Overall, a gluten-free diet, when properly managed, can offer substantial health benefits and an enhanced sense of well-being for those sensitive to gluten.

HOW TO IDENTIFY GLUTEN

Understanding gluten content through ratings involves reading food labels and relying on certification symbols. Look for labels that explicitly state "gluten-free" to ensure the product meets regulatory standards. Additionally, certifications like the Gluten-Free Certification Organization (GFCO) or the Certified Gluten-Free label signify compliance with specific gluten thresholds. Some products display a star-rating system or numerical indications to denote gluten content, where a lower number or fewer stars implies lower gluten levels. However, always prioritize labels explicitly stating "gluten-free" or certified by reputable organizations to reliably identify gluten-free products and ensure they meet your dietary requirements.

HOW TO USE THIS FOOD LIST

Using a gluten-free food list involves several steps:

1. Familiarize Yourself: Review the list thoroughly to understand the various categories and types of foods that are gluten-free.

2. Check Ingredients: When shopping, examine product labels for ingredients. Cross-reference against the food list to ensure items don't contain gluten or its derivatives.

3. Meal Planning: Incorporate the listed gluten-free foods into your meal plans. Create recipes using gluten-free grains, vegetables, proteins, and snacks from the list.

4. Explore Alternatives: Use the list to discover gluten-free substitutes for traditional gluten-containing items. For instance, try quinoa or rice pasta instead of wheat-based pasta.

. Dining Out: Refer to the list when eating out. Look for restaurants offering gluten-free options or dishes that align with the listed foods.

. Stay Updated: As new products hit the market or food trends change, keep the list current. Update it with new gluten-free finds or alternatives.

. Share Knowledge: If you have friends or family with gluten sensitivities, share the list to help them navigate their dietary needs.

Remember, while the list serves as a helpful guide, always double-check labels for any changes in ingredients or manufacturing processes. Over time, your familiarity with these foods will make shopping and meal planning more intuitive.

GRAINS AND FLOURS

"Grains and Flours" in the context of gluten-free eating offer a diverse range of alternatives to traditional wheat-based options. Quinoa, rice, millet, and buckwheat are versatile gluten-free grains that can be used in various dishes, from pilafs to baking. These grains not only provide a different taste and texture but also offer nutritional benefits like higher protein content and essential vitamins and minerals.

When it comes to flours, almond, coconut, chickpea, and tapioca flours are popular gluten-free substitutes. They serve as excellent options for baking, thickening sauces, or creating gluten-free coatings for frying. Understanding the properties of each flour helps in choosing the right one for specific recipes, maintaining texture and taste while avoiding gluten.

Exploring these gluten-free grains and flours opens up a world of culinary possibilities, allowing individuals on a gluten-free diet to enjoy a wide array of delicious and nutritious meals without compromising taste or quality.

RICE

Rice stands out as a versatile and naturally gluten-free grain, making it a staple for those following a gluten-free diet. Its inherent lack of gluten—found abundantly in wheat, barley, and rye—makes rice a safe and essential component in gluten-free meal plans. Whether it's white, brown, black, jasmine, or basmati, all varieties of rice are inherently devoid of gluten, providing a safe carbohydrate option.

This grain offers culinary flexibility, allowing for diverse meal creations. From rice bowls and risottos to sushi and rice flour used in gluten-free baking, its adaptability in various cuisines worldwide ensures those with gluten sensitivities have ample choices. Its neutral taste also blends seamlessly with other flavors, enhancing its appeal in gluten-free cooking. Due to its prevalence and safety for those avoiding gluten, rice stands as a reliable and widely embraced component in gluten-free diets, offering both nutritional value and gastronomic delight.

QUINOA

Quinoa, pronounced keen-wah, is a gluten-free ancient grain celebrated for its nutritional prowess and versatility in the kitchen. As a naturally gluten-free whole grain, quinoa stands as a valuable staple for those adhering to a gluten-free diet due to celiac disease or gluten sensitivity.

Rich in essential nutrients like fiber, iron, magnesium, and various vitamins, quinoa offers a wholesome substitute for gluten-containing grains. Its nutty flavor and slightly chewy texture make it an excellent ingredient for salads, soups, stir-fries, and even as a breakfast porridge. Quinoa's adaptability allows it to be used as a base for gluten-free pasta, flour, or as a standalone side dish.

Moreover, its complete protein profile, containing all nine essential amino acids, makes quinoa a particularly valuable addition to vegetarian or vegan diets. Its gluten-free nature and impressive nutritional content have contributed to its popularity as a nutritious, gluten-free alternative in various culinary applications.

BUCKWHEAT

Buckwheat, despite its name, isn't a wheat variety and is naturally gluten-free. It's a nutritious pseudo-cereal that serves as an excellent alternative for those avoiding gluten. This triangular seed, when ground into flour, becomes a versatile ingredient suitable for various recipes, including pancakes, noodles, and baked goods.

Rich in essential nutrients like fiber, protein, vitamins, and minerals such as magnesium and iron, buckwheat offers numerous health benefits. Its high fiber content aids digestion and promotes a feeling of fullness, while its impressive protein profile makes it a valuable addition to a plant-based or gluten-free diet.

Due to its gluten-free nature, buckwheat is a popular choice for individuals with celiac disease, gluten sensitivities, or those simply looking to diversify their diet with wholesome, gluten-free grains. Incorporating buckwheat into meals not only adds a unique nutty flavor but also contributes to a balanced and nutritious gluten-free eating plan.

CORNMEAL

Cornmeal is a gluten-free staple made from ground maize. Its naturally gluten-free composition makes it an excellent alternative for those avoiding gluten due to celiac disease or gluten sensitivity. This coarse flour boasts versatility in cooking, used in various culinary traditions worldwide. From classic cornbread to tortillas, tamales, and polenta, cornmeal serves as a foundational ingredient in numerous dishes.

Beyond its culinary appeal, cornmeal offers nutritional benefits. It's rich in fiber, antioxidants, and essential minerals like magnesium and phosphorus. This nutrient profile contributes to digestive health, aids in regular bowel movements, and supports overall well-being. Additionally, cornmeal's distinct texture and mild flavor enhance both sweet and savory recipes, making it a valuable addition to gluten-free diets and a go-to ingredient for creating delicious, gluten-free meals without compromising taste or texture.

ALMOND FLOUR

Almond flour, made from finely ground almonds, stands out as a versatile and gluten-free alternative to traditional wheat-based flours. Its natural lack of gluten makes it an ideal choice for those following a gluten-free diet due to celiac disease, gluten intolerance, or preference.

This flour boasts a subtly sweet, nutty flavor, adding richness to baked goods like cookies, cakes, and muffins. Almond flour's moisture-retaining properties contribute to moist and tender textures in recipes. Its high protein and healthy fat content also offer nutritional benefits, aiding in satiety and providing essential nutrients like vitamin E and magnesium.

For those seeking to replace wheat flour in recipes, almond flour often requires adjustments due to its different texture and moisture absorption. It's a common choice in grain-free and paleo diets as well. Incorporating almond flour not only accommodates gluten-free needs but also introduces a nutritious and flavorful element to various culinary creations.

COCONUT FLOUR

Coconut flour stands out in the realm of gluten-free alternatives due to its natural absence of gluten. Derived from dried coconut meat, this flour is a versatile and nutritious option for those on a gluten-free diet. Not only does it lack gluten, but it's also high in fiber, protein, and healthy fats, making it a wholesome choice for baking and cooking.

Its ability to absorb moisture differently from traditional flours requires adjustments in recipes, often needing more liquid or eggs to achieve the desired consistency. When used in baking, coconut flour lends a subtly sweet, tropical flavor to dishes, elevating the taste profile. It's an excellent option for creating gluten-free baked goods like muffins, pancakes, and even bread.

Overall, coconut flour's gluten-free nature, coupled with its nutritional benefits and unique flavor, makes it a valuable ingredient for those seeking alternative flours in their gluten-free culinary adventures.

VEGETABLES AND FRUITS

"Vegetables and Fruits" form a cornerstone of a gluten-free diet, offering an array of naturally safe options. These whole foods are inherently free of gluten, making them an essential part of meals for those with celiac disease or gluten sensitivities. From leafy greens like spinach and kale to vibrant fruits like berries and citrus, the variety available ensures a diverse and nutritious diet.

Incorporating a spectrum of colors ensures a rich intake of vitamins, minerals, and antioxidants, supporting overall health. Whether consumed raw, cooked, or as ingredients in gluten-free recipes, vegetables and fruits provide fiber for digestive health while offering a range of flavors and textures. Their versatility allows for endless culinary creativity, enabling individuals to craft delicious and gluten-free meals easily. When exploring a gluten-free lifestyle, these natural, unprocessed options from the "Vegetables and Fruits" category become foundational for a well-rounded, healthy diet.

FRESH PRODUCE

Fresh produce inherently comprises gluten-free options, offering a wide array of nutritious choices for those following a gluten-free diet. Fruits and vegetables, whether organic or conventionally grown, are naturally devoid of gluten, making them safe for consumption.

Including ample fresh produce in a gluten-free diet ensures a rich source of vitamins, minerals, antioxidants, and dietary fiber. Colorful fruits like berries, oranges, and apples, along with vegetables such as leafy greens, bell peppers, and carrots, not only provide essential nutrients but also offer versatility in meal preparation.

Incorporating fresh produce into gluten-free meals can enhance flavor, texture, and nutritional value. From vibrant salads to hearty stir-fries and smoothies, the variety and nutritional benefits of fresh fruits and vegetables play a pivotal role in maintaining a balanced and healthy gluten-free lifestyle.

CANNED OR FROZEN OPTIONS

Canned or frozen options can be a convenient and reliable choice for those following a gluten-free diet. When selecting canned goods or frozen items, it's essential to scrutinize labels for any added ingredients that might contain gluten. Many companies now explicitly mark their products as gluten-free, offering peace of mind to consumers.

Canned vegetables, fruits (in natural juices or water), and legumes are often gluten-free, but it's wise to avoid items with added sauces or seasonings unless they're explicitly labeled gluten-free. Similarly, frozen vegetables, fruits, and seafood without any added coatings or sauces are typically safe choices for a gluten-free diet.

Always verify the packaging for any potential cross-contamination risks, especially in shared manufacturing facilities. With the right attention to labels and ingredients, canned or frozen options can serve as versatile staples in crafting delicious and safe gluten-free meals.

PROTEINS

The protein category in a gluten-free food list encompasses various options that offer essential nutrients without containing gluten. These protein sources are crucial for maintaining muscle health, supporting bodily functions, and providing sustained energy. Gluten-free protein sources range from animal-based products like poultry, fish, beef, and eggs to plant-based alternatives such as legumes (like lentils and chickpeas), nuts, seeds, and tofu. Each of these sources offers its unique set of amino acids, vitamins, and minerals necessary for overall well-being.

When following a gluten-free diet, individuals often rely on these diverse protein sources to ensure they meet their nutritional needs without inadvertently consuming gluten. These proteins serve as versatile ingredients in meal preparation, allowing for a wide array of recipes and culinary creations. Understanding and incorporating these gluten-free protein options into daily meals not only ensures a balanced diet but also contributes to dietary variety and can cater to different dietary preferences or restrictions beyond gluten sensitivity or celiac disease. Incorporating a range of gluten-free proteins allows for a diverse and satisfying diet while steering clear of gluten-containing products.

MEAT

The protein category in a gluten-free food list encompasses various options that offer essential nutrients without containing gluten. These protein sources are crucial for maintaining muscle health, supporting bodily functions, and providing sustained energy. Gluten-free protein sources range from animal-based products like poultry, fish, beef, and eggs to plant-based alternatives such as legumes (like lentils and chickpeas), nuts, seeds, and tofu. Each of these sources offers its unique set of amino acids, vitamins, and minerals necessary for overall well-being.

When following a gluten-free diet, individuals often rely on these diverse protein sources to ensure they meet their nutritional needs without inadvertently consuming gluten. These proteins serve as versatile ingredients in meal preparation, allowing for a wide array of recipes and culinary creations. Understanding and incorporating these gluten-free protein options into daily meals not only ensures a balanced diet but also contributes to dietary variety and can cater to different dietary preferences or restrictions beyond gluten sensitivity or celiac disease. Incorporating a range of gluten-free proteins allows for a diverse and satisfying diet while steering clear of gluten-containing products.

FISH AND SEAFOOD

Fish and seafood are naturally gluten-free, making them excellent choices for those following a gluten-free diet. These protein-rich options include a vast array of choices, from salmon and tuna to shrimp, mussels, and more. Whether fresh, frozen, or canned, most fish and seafood are free from gluten additives or cross-contamination.

However, caution is advised with processed or breaded seafood items, as they might contain gluten in their coatings or added ingredients. When buying pre-marinated or seasoned seafood, it's essential to check the labels for any gluten-containing additives or sauces.

For a safe and gluten-free dining experience, opt for fresh cuts or ask about preparation methods when dining out. Grilling, baking, or sautéing seafood using gluten-free ingredients and avoiding shared cooking surfaces can ensure delicious and safe gluten-free meals. Fish and seafood provide versatile and healthy options for those following a gluten-free lifestyle, offering abundant nutritional benefits without the worry of gluten content.

LEGUMES AND BEANS

Legumes and beans are naturally gluten-free, offering a versatile and nutritious option for those following a gluten-free diet. These protein-packed foods, including lentils, chickpeas, black beans, and peas, serve as excellent alternatives to gluten-containing grains. They are rich in fiber, vitamins, and minerals while being inherently free from gluten, making them a staple for individuals with celiac disease or gluten sensitivity.

These legumes and beans can be incorporated into various dishes, from soups and stews to salads and main courses. They provide a satisfying texture and can even be ground into flours for gluten-free baking. Their versatility and nutritional profile make them essential components of a balanced gluten-free diet, offering not just a substitute for gluten-containing grains but also contributing to a diverse and flavorful culinary experience.

TOFU AND TEMPEH

Tofu and tempeh are naturally gluten-free plant-based protein sources, offering versatile and nutritious options for those on a gluten-free diet. Both are derived from soybeans but undergo different fermentation processes.

Tofu, made by coagulating soy milk, is inherently gluten-free. It's a versatile ingredient that can be used in various cuisines and dishes, providing a good source of protein, iron, and calcium.

Tempeh, another soy-based product, results from fermenting whole soybeans. This fermentation process can enhance nutrient absorption and digestibility. Like tofu, tempeh is gluten-free, providing a meaty texture and a nutty flavor profile. It's rich in protein, probiotics, and other essential nutrients.

When incorporating tofu or tempeh into a gluten-free diet, ensure any marinades or sauces used in recipes are also gluten-free. These soy-based products serve as excellent meat alternatives, contributing to a well-rounded and flavorful gluten-free meal plan.

DAIRY AND ALTERNATIVES

"Dairy and Alternatives" within a gluten-free context encompass various milk products and substitutes devoid of gluten. While dairy itself doesn't contain gluten, cross-contamination can occur in flavored or processed dairy items. Always opt for plain, unflavored dairy products like milk, yogurt, and cheese, checking labels for any added ingredients that might contain gluten.

For those lactose intolerant or seeking non-dairy options, numerous gluten-free alternatives exist. Almond, coconut, soy, and rice milk are popular dairy substitutes. When choosing dairy alternatives, scrutinize labels to ensure they're explicitly labeled "gluten-free," as some may contain thickeners or flavorings derived from gluten sources. Additionally, several plant-based cheeses and yogurts, made from ingredients like nuts, seeds, or tofu, offer gluten-free options. Being vigilant about ingredients and certifications ensures that dairy or its substitutes align with a gluten-free diet, catering to diverse dietary preferences and restrictions.

MILK SUBSTITUTES

Milk substitutes are a vital component of a gluten-free diet, especially for individuals with lactose intolerance or those seeking dairy alternatives. Many milk substitutes inherently do not contain gluten, offering safe options for those sensitive to this protein. Common gluten-free milk alternatives include almond milk, coconut milk, soy milk, oat milk, and rice milk.

It's essential to verify the ingredients on packaged milk substitutes, as some flavored or fortified versions might contain gluten additives. Opt for products explicitly labeled as "gluten-free" or certified by reliable organizations to ensure they meet gluten safety standards. These alternatives not only cater to dietary restrictions but also provide essential nutrients like calcium and vitamin D, offering a versatile range of options for beverages, cooking, and baking without compromising on taste or nutritional value for individuals adhering to a gluten-free lifestyle.

CHEESE ALTERNATIVES

Cheese alternatives, crafted for those following a gluten-free diet, offer a diverse array of options. Many cheeses inherently lack gluten, but certain flavored or processed varieties might contain additives that could introduce gluten. Opting for natural, unprocessed cheeses like cheddar, mozzarella, Swiss, or goat cheese ensures a gluten-free choice.

Moreover, the market now offers plant-based alternatives like almond, cashew, or soy-based cheeses explicitly labeled gluten-free. These dairy-free options not only cater to individuals with lactose intolerance but also suit those avoiding gluten. Checking labels is crucial, as some dairy-free cheeses may contain gluten-based thickeners or flavor enhancers.

When incorporating cheese alternatives into recipes or meals, verify their gluten-free status and explore different types to diversify flavors and textures. Whether for melting on pizzas, topping salads, or creating dairy-free cheese sauces, these alternatives provide flexibility and delicious options for those adhering to a gluten-free lifestyle.

YOGURT ALTERNATIVES

Yogurt alternatives offer a diverse range of options for those following a gluten-free diet. Traditional yogurt might contain additives or thickeners that contain gluten, posing a risk for those sensitive to it. However, numerous gluten-free alternatives cater to various dietary needs.

Plant-based yogurts derived from coconut, almond, soy, or oats are often naturally gluten-free and serve as excellent alternatives. They offer similar creamy textures and come in various flavors, providing versatility in culinary applications and dietary preferences.

Checking labels is crucial, as some yogurt alternatives may contain gluten-based additives for texture or flavor. Opt for products clearly labeled "gluten-free" to ensure they meet dietary requirements. Additionally, homemade yogurt using gluten-free ingredients offers a customizable and wholesome option for those seeking complete control over their diet. Overall, exploring yogurt alternatives opens up a world of gluten-free options without compromising taste or nutritional value.

SNACKS AND TREATS

"Snacks and Treats" within the realm of gluten-free options offer a diverse array of delicious choices that cater to varying preferences and dietary needs. These options ensure those with gluten sensitivities or celiac disease can still indulge in delightful snacks without compromising their health.

Nuts and seeds stand out as versatile and nutritious options. They're naturally gluten-free and provide a satisfying crunch, making them ideal for snacking. Additionally, gluten-free snack bars, made from ingredients like nuts, dried fruits, and gluten-free grains such as quinoa or oats, offer convenient and flavorful choices. These bars come in various flavors and are often formulated to provide sustained energy.

Popcorn, when not seasoned with gluten-containing flavorings, is an excellent gluten-free snack. Its light and airy texture make it enjoyable while being a whole grain option. Rice cakes, too, are a versatile base for sweet or savory toppings and are inherently gluten-free.

Exploring the world of gluten-free snacks and treats also involves discovering dedicated gluten-free versions of traditional favorites. Companies now produce gluten-free cookies, cakes, and brownies using alternative flours like almond or coconut flour, allowing individuals to savor familiar treats without gluten-related concerns.

Overall, the gluten-free snack landscape is diverse, offering both nutritious and indulgent options, making it easier for individuals to maintain a gluten-free lifestyle without sacrificing flavor or variety.

NUTS AND SEEDS

Nuts and seeds are excellent additions to a gluten-free diet. Naturally free from gluten, they offer a versatile and nutritious range of options. These nutrient-dense foods provide healthy fats, protein, fiber, vitamins, and minerals, making them valuable for those adhering to a gluten-free lifestyle.

Options like almonds, walnuts, pecans, and pistachios offer a satisfying crunch and are perfect for snacking or incorporating into meals. They serve as fantastic gluten-free alternatives for traditional processed snacks that might contain gluten.

Seeds such as chia, flaxseed, sunflower seeds, and pumpkin seeds are also gluten-free powerhouses. They can be sprinkled on salads, added to smoothies, or used in baking as substitutes for gluten-containing ingredients, offering texture, flavor, and a nutritional boost.

However, while nuts and seeds themselves are naturally gluten-free, caution is advised when purchasing flavored or seasoned varieties. Some commercially seasoned nuts or seeds might contain gluten-based additives in their flavorings, so it's crucial to read labels carefully to ensure they're free from gluten or any cross-contamination.

Overall, nuts and seeds are not only gluten-free staples but also provide a healthy array of nutrients, offering a delicious and diverse range of options for those following a gluten-free diet.

GLUTEN-FREE SNACK BARS

Gluten-free snack bars offer a convenient and tasty solution for individuals seeking gluten-free options while on the go. These bars are crafted without gluten-containing ingredients like wheat, barley, or rye, making them suitable for those with celiac disease or gluten sensitivity. They often feature alternative grains like rice, quinoa, or certified gluten-free oats as a base, providing a satisfying texture and taste without compromising dietary restrictions.

These bars come in a variety of flavors and types, from nut-based to fruit-infused options, catering to different preferences and nutritional needs. They're not just a handy snack; they often contain a mix of proteins, healthy fats, and fiber, offering a balanced nutritional profile ideal for a quick energy boost between meals.

When selecting gluten-free snack bars, it's essential to check labels for gluten-free certifications or explicitly stated gluten-free claims. While many brands cater to gluten-free diets, cross-contamination remains a concern, emphasizing the importance of confirming the absence of gluten traces in the manufacturing process.

Gluten-free snack bars serve as a versatile option for those managing gluten-related disorders, providing a portable, safe, and delicious snack choice that aligns with their dietary requirements, ensuring they can enjoy a convenient treat without compromising their health.

POPCORN

Popcorn is a naturally gluten-free whole grain snack, making it a safe and enjoyable option for those following a gluten-free diet. As long as it's not processed with gluten-containing additives or seasonings, popcorn retains its gluten-free status. This simple yet versatile snack can be air-popped or prepared using minimal oil on the stovetop, allowing for various flavoring options.

However, it's essential to be cautious when consuming pre-packaged or flavored popcorn varieties, as additives, seasonings, or coatings might introduce gluten. Always check the labels for any potential gluten ingredients, especially in flavored or microwave popcorn options. Opting for plain, unadorned popcorn kernels or those explicitly labeled as gluten-free ensures a safe choice.

Popcorn is not just a delicious snack; it also offers nutritional benefits. It's a good source of fiber, antioxidants, and whole grains, contributing to digestive health and providing a satisfying crunch without the gluten content found in many other snacks. Whether enjoyed at home or purchased from a trusted source, popcorn stands out as a convenient, naturally gluten-free snack option for individuals adhering to gluten-free dietary restrictions.

RICE CAKES

Rice cakes serve as a popular gluten-free alternative to various wheat-based snacks. These light and crunchy snacks are typically made from puffed rice and offer a versatile base for both sweet and savory toppings. One of the primary advantages of rice cakes is their inherent gluten-free nature, making them suitable for individuals with celiac disease or gluten sensitivities.

As they're crafted primarily from rice, a naturally gluten-free grain, rice cakes pose minimal risk of gluten contamination, provided they're not processed in facilities that handle gluten-containing ingredients. Their gluten-free status makes them a convenient option for snacking or as a substitute for bread in various recipes.

Moreover, rice cakes come in an array of flavors, from plain to multigrain or infused with seasonings like sea salt, cinnamon, or even chocolate coatings. Toppings such as nut butter, avocado, or hummus complement their neutral taste, offering endless possibilities for customization.

Their compact size and shelf-stable nature make rice cakes a convenient on-the-go snack option. However, it's essential to check packaging labels to ensure the absence of gluten-containing additives or cross-contamination, especially if you have severe gluten-related disorders. Overall, rice cakes stand as a versatile and naturally gluten-free snack, catering to diverse dietary preferences and needs.

CONDIMENTS AND SAUCES

Condiments and sauces can be tricky areas when adhering to a gluten-free diet. Gluten often hides in these products as a thickening agent or flavor enhancer. When exploring gluten-free options in this category, it's crucial to scrutinize labels thoroughly. Look for products explicitly labeled as "gluten-free" to ensure they meet safety standards. Additionally, ingredients like wheat, barley, or rye should be absent from the list to guarantee the condiment or sauce is safe for consumption.

Some condiments naturally steer clear of gluten, such as mustard or certain types of vinegar. However, items like soy sauce, hoisin sauce, or some gravies frequently contain gluten unless specified otherwise. Awareness of alternative ingredients used in gluten-free versions of condiments, such as cornstarch or rice flour for thickening, is beneficial.

Opting for homemade versions of condiments allows for complete control over ingredients, ensuring they align with a gluten-free diet. Finally, when dining out or using unfamiliar brands, don't hesitate to inquire about ingredients or preparation methods to safeguard against accidental gluten exposure. Understanding the nuances of condiments and sauces in relation to gluten is essential for maintaining a gluten-free lifestyle.

SALAD DRESSINGS

Salad dressings, while seemingly innocent, can often hide gluten-containing ingredients like wheat-based thickeners or malt vinegar. Opting for gluten-free salad dressings is crucial for those following a gluten-free diet. Fortunately, many brands offer explicitly labeled gluten-free options.

Look for dressings labeled "gluten-free" to ensure they don't contain any hidden gluten sources. Ingredients like cornstarch, rice vinegar, or tamari (gluten-free soy sauce) are commonly used in gluten-free dressings as alternatives to wheat-based additives. Homemade dressings using gluten-free ingredients like olive oil, balsamic vinegar, lemon juice, and herbs can also ensure a safe gluten-free option.

When dining out or purchasing pre-made dressings, always ask about ingredients or look for allergen information on labels. Being vigilant about salad dressings is essential in maintaining a gluten-free diet and enjoying salads without the risk of gluten-related reactions, ensuring a safe and enjoyable dining experience.

SALSAS AND DIPS

Salsas and dips offer flavorful accompaniments to meals, but for individuals following a gluten-free diet, it's crucial to navigate these options carefully. Most homemade salsas, guacamole, hummus, and bean dips are naturally gluten-free, relying on ingredients like tomatoes, avocados, beans, and herbs. However, store-bought varieties might include additives or thickeners that contain gluten.

To ensure a gluten-free choice, read labels attentively. Look for "gluten-free" labeling or certifications. Corn-based tortilla chips, fresh vegetable sticks, or rice crackers serve as excellent gluten-free dipping options. Consider making homemade salsas or dips using fresh ingredients to guarantee they're free from gluten-containing additives.

Popular dips like queso or cheese-based varieties may contain gluten if thickeners or flavorings are added. Always check ingredient lists or consider preparing these dips from scratch using gluten-free ingredients. By exercising caution and being aware of ingredients, enjoying gluten-free salsas and dips can be a flavorful and worry-free experience.

GLUTEN-FREE SOY SAUCE ALTERNATIVES

For individuals on a gluten-free diet, traditional soy sauce poses a challenge as it contains wheat, a gluten-containing grain. However, several gluten-free soy sauce alternatives cater to these dietary restrictions. Tamari, often considered a gluten-free substitute, is a Japanese soy sauce made without wheat and exclusively from soybeans. It maintains a rich umami flavor, perfect for seasoning various dishes.

Coconut aminos, derived from coconut sap, offer a sweeter and milder alternative to soy sauce. This option is not only gluten-free but also soy-free, making it suitable for those with multiple dietary restrictions. Additionally, there are commercial brands that specifically produce gluten-free soy sauce, clearly labeled to indicate their compliance with gluten-free standards.

These alternatives provide individuals adhering to a gluten-free diet with flavorful options for seasoning and enhancing the taste of their meals without compromising their dietary needs.

BEVERAGES

Gluten-free beverages encompass a wide range of options suitable for those with gluten sensitivities or celiac disease. Natural choices like water, coffee, and tea are inherently gluten-free. Fruit juices, including fresh-squeezed or packaged varieties without additives, are also safe.

When considering alcoholic beverages, many spirits like vodka, gin, tequila, and rum are typically gluten-free as the distillation process removes gluten proteins. However, flavored or malted alcoholic drinks, beer, and some specialty cocktails may contain gluten. Opting for gluten-free beer, cider, or distilled beverages marked as gluten-free ensures a safe choice.

Additionally, exploring alternative milk options such as almond, coconut, soy, or oat milk can provide gluten-free substitutes for individuals who are lactose intolerant or prefer non-dairy beverages.

Always check labels or opt for products labeled "gluten-free" to ensure these beverages align with your dietary needs, offering a refreshing array of choices while keeping gluten at bay.

COFFEE AND TEA

Coffee and tea, in their pure forms, are naturally gluten-free, making them safe options for those following a gluten-free diet. However, potential gluten contamination can occur through flavorings, additives, or cross-contact during processing and preparation.

Some flavored or specialty coffee and tea blends may contain additives that include gluten-based ingredients. It's essential to check labels and opt for products explicitly labeled "gluten-free" to ensure safety. Additionally, when ordering coffee or tea from cafes or shops, inquire about potential cross-contamination risks from shared equipment or preparation surfaces.

Choosing single-origin coffees or pure tea leaves minimizes the likelihood of gluten exposure. Most unadulterated coffee beans and tea leaves maintain their gluten-free status, allowing individuals with gluten sensitivities to enjoy these beverages without concern. Being vigilant about ingredients and production processes guarantees a safe gluten-free experience when indulging in coffee or tea.

FRUIT JUICES

Fruit juices are naturally gluten-free as they're derived purely from fruits without any added gluten-containing ingredients. Whether freshly squeezed or commercially produced, fruit juices typically do not contain gluten. However, cross-contamination could occur during processing or packaging if the facility handles gluten-containing products.

To ensure a juice is gluten-free, it's crucial to check labels or contact the manufacturer, especially for blended or flavored juices. Some companies might use additives or additional ingredients that could introduce gluten. Look for clear labeling indicating "gluten-free" or certifications from recognized gluten-free organizations to guarantee the absence of gluten in fruit juices. Opting for freshly squeezed juices or those explicitly labeled gluten-free provides a safe and enjoyable choice for individuals following a gluten-free diet, allowing them to relish the natural flavors of various fruits without concerns about gluten contamination.

ALCOHOLIC BEVERAGES

When it comes to alcoholic beverages and gluten, it's essential to choose wisely for a gluten-free diet. Certain alcoholic drinks are naturally gluten-free, while others may contain gluten due to their production process.

Options like wine, pure distilled liquors (such as vodka, gin, and tequila), and most hard ciders are generally safe for a gluten-free diet. During distillation, gluten proteins typically do not carry over into the final product, making these spirits safe for many with gluten sensitivity.

However, it's crucial to be cautious with beers, as most traditional beers are brewed using gluten-containing grains like barley, wheat, or rye. Thankfully, the market offers an expanding selection of gluten-free beers brewed with alternative grains like sorghum, rice, or millet, catering to those avoiding gluten.

Always check labels or do some research on specific brands to ensure their alcoholic beverages are gluten-free, especially if gluten sensitivity is a concern.

EATING OUT AND GLUTEN-FREE OPTIONS

Navigating gluten-free options while dining out requires some savvy and communication. Here's a comprehensive guide to ensure a safe and enjoyable experience:

1. Research and Choose Wisely: Before heading out, research restaurants known for accommodating gluten-free diets. Check their menus online or call ahead to inquire about gluten-free offerings.

2. Communicate Clearly: Upon arrival, inform your server about your gluten-free requirements. Clearly articulate your needs, emphasizing the importance of avoiding gluten due to health reasons.

3. Grill on Ingredients and Preparation: Ask detailed questions about how dishes are prepared. Inquire about ingredients, potential cross-contamination risks, and if the kitchen has protocols for gluten-free meals.

4. Identify Safe Options: Many restaurants mark gluten-free items on their menu or have separate gluten-free menus. Focus on naturally gluten-free

choices like salads, grilled meats, seafood, or dishes made with rice or quinoa.

5. Beware of Hidden Gluten: Sauces, marinades, and seasonings often contain gluten. Request these on the side or ask for alternatives to ensure a gluten-free meal.

6. Be Wary of Cross-Contamination: Even if a dish seems gluten-free, cross-contamination in the kitchen can occur. Request separate utensils or cooking surfaces to prevent contact with gluten-containing foods.

7. Stay Vigilant: Despite your efforts, mistakes can happen. Trust your instincts and if unsure, don't hesitate to ask more questions or choose a different dish.

8. Express Gratitude: Acknowledge and thank the staff for their attention to your dietary needs. It encourages restaurants to continue providing gluten-free options and raises awareness among their team.

By being proactive, communicative, and vigilant, dining out gluten-free can be a safe and enjoyable experience. Research, communication, and a little caution can help ensure a pleasant meal without compromising your dietary needs.

GLUTEN-FREE FOOD LIST DICTIONARY

RATING SYSTEM

0 = No Gluten

1 = possibility of Gluten (depending on make or production)

2 = High chance of Gluten

3 = Highest possibility of Gluten (these should be completely avoided)

Apple

Apples are naturally gluten-free, earning a "0" on the gluten rating scale. This fruit is a wholesome choice for those following a gluten-free diet, offering fiber, vitamins, and antioxidants without any gluten-related concerns. Whether enjoyed fresh, sliced into salads, or used in gluten-free baking, apples stand as a versatile and safe option for individuals managing gluten sensitivities or celiac disease.

Rating : 0

Alcohol

When it comes to alcohol, it's essential for those on a gluten-free diet to be vigilant. Distilled spirits like vodka, gin, and rum are generally considered gluten-free, as the distillation process removes gluten. However, beer and malt-based beverages contain gluten. Opt for certified gluten-free beers or naturally gluten-free options like wine and most distilled liquors.

Rating : 2

Avocado

Avocado is a naturally gluten-free fruit, scoring a definitive zero on the gluten rating scale. Rich in healthy fats, fiber, vitamins, and minerals, avocados are a versatile addition to a gluten-free diet. Whether sliced on toast or used in salads, dips, or smoothies, avocados are a nutrient-dense and delicious option for those seeking gluten-free, wholesome foods.

Rating : 0

Banana

Bananas are naturally gluten-free, containing no gluten proteins. They're a nutritious fruit packed with potassium, vitamins, and fiber, making them a fantastic addition to a gluten-free diet. Bananas score a perfect "zero" on the gluten rating scale, ensuring they're safe for those with celiac disease or gluten sensitivities. Enjoyed on their own, in smoothies, or used as a versatile ingredient in gluten-free baking, bananas are a wholesome and safe choice.

Rating : 0

Blueberries

Blueberries are naturally gluten-free, containing no measurable amounts of gluten. These small, flavorful fruits are rich in antioxidants, vitamins, and fiber, offering numerous health benefits. Whether consumed fresh, frozen, or incorporated into various dishes like smoothies, salads, or baked goods, blueberries are a safe and nutritious choice for those adhering to a gluten-free diet. They're a delicious addition to meals without posing any risks for gluten-related concerns.

Rating : 0

Bagel

Bagels, traditional wheat-based delights, unfortunately contain gluten due to their composition of wheat flour. This beloved round bread, while a breakfast staple, poses a risk for individuals sensitive to gluten. Gluten content in bagels makes them unsuitable for those with celiac disease or gluten intolerance. However, there are gluten-free bagel alternatives available, typically crafted using alternative flours like rice or almond flour, ensuring a safe option for those adhering to a gluten-free diet.

Rating : 3

Banana

Bananas are naturally gluten-free, scoring a perfect 0 on the gluten rating scale. These nutritious fruits are packed with vitamins, minerals, and dietary fiber. Being naturally gluten-free makes them a safe and versatile choice for those with celiac disease or gluten sensitivities. Bananas serve as a delicious snack, a natural sweetener in baked goods, and a versatile ingredient in smoothies, adding both flavor and valuable nutrients to various dishes.

Rating : 0

Beans

Beans, including black beans, kidney beans, and chickpeas, are inherently gluten-free. They're versatile, protein-packed staples often used in gluten-free diets. Rich in fiber and nutrients, they're rated gluten-free, making them an excellent choice for those with celiac disease or gluten sensitivity seeking safe and nutritious options.

Rating : 0

Beef

Beef is naturally gluten-free, providing a rich source of protein and essential nutrients. Whether grilled, roasted, or stewed, it remains a safe option for those following a gluten-free diet. To ensure gluten-free status, seasonings, marinades, and sauces should be checked for potential gluten-containing ingredients.

Rating : 1

Beetroot

Beetroot, a nutrient-rich root vegetable packed with antioxidants, vitamins, and minerals, boasts a naturally gluten-free status. Its vibrant color and earthy flavor make it a versatile ingredient in gluten-free diets. From salads to smoothies, beetroot offers culinary flexibility without any gluten concerns. This wholesome vegetable's nutritional benefits, combined with its gluten-free nature, make it a valuable addition to a balanced and diverse diet.

Rating : 0

Blackberry

Blackberries are naturally gluten-free, making them a safe choice for those with gluten-related sensitivities. Packed with antioxidants, vitamins, and fiber, these flavorful berries contribute to a healthy diet. Whether enjoyed fresh, frozen, or incorporated into various dishes like smoothies, salads, or desserts, blackberries offer a delicious and nutritious addition without any gluten concerns, allowing everyone to savor their benefits worry-free.

Rating : 0

Blueberry

Blackberries are vibrant, nutrient-rich fruits known for their sweet-tart flavor and numerous health benefits. They're naturally gluten-free, making them a safe choice for those following a gluten-free diet. Packed with antioxidants, vitamins C and K, and dietary fiber, blackberries contribute to a healthy immune system and digestive health. Their low gluten content, essentially gluten-free status, makes them a versatile and delicious addition to various dishes and snacks.

Rating : 0

Broccoli

Broccoli, a nutrient-packed cruciferous vegetable, boasts a naturally gluten-free profile. This versatile veggie is rich in vitamins, fiber, and antioxidants, offering numerous health benefits. Its gluten rating is 0, making it an excellent choice for those adhering to a gluten-free diet. Whether steamed, roasted, or added to various dishes, broccoli stands out as a flavorful and safe option for gluten-sensitive individuals seeking nutritious meal options.

Rating : 0

Brussels Sprouts

Brussels sprouts, a nutrient-packed cruciferous vegetable, are naturally gluten-free. These miniature cabbages are rich in vitamins K and C, fiber, and antioxidants, contributing to a healthy diet. With zero gluten, they're a safe and versatile choice for gluten-sensitive individuals. Whether roasted, sautéed, or steamed, Brussels sprouts offer a delicious way to add nutritional value to meals without any concern for gluten content.

Rating : 0

Burger

Indulge in a juicy burger without worries about gluten. Opt for a gluten-free bun or wrap your savory patty in lettuce for a satisfying crunch. Season your ground beef, turkey, or plant-based burger with gluten-free spices and herbs. Top it off with fresh vegetables, cheese, and condiments marked as gluten-free. Ensure a worry-free meal by checking for gluten-free labels on all ingredients to enjoy your burger guilt-free.

Rating : 2

Cabbage

Cabbage is a naturally gluten-free vegetable with a high nutritional value. Rich in vitamins K, C, and B, it offers antioxidants and fiber beneficial for gut health. Being naturally gluten-free, cabbage has no gluten proteins. It's versatile for various diets, making it an excellent addition for those avoiding gluten. Incorporate it into salads, stir-fries, or fermented dishes like sauerkraut for a flavorful, gluten-free option in meals.

Rating : 0

Cantaloupe

Cantaloupe, a delicious and juicy melon, naturally earns a "gluten-free" rating. Rich in vitamins A and C, this hydrating fruit is low in calories and high in dietary fiber, aiding digestion. Its sweet, orange flesh provides a refreshing treat while delivering essential nutrients. Being naturally gluten-free, cantaloupe makes for a safe and enjoyable choice for those following a gluten-free diet, offering a guilt-free, nutritious snack or addition to meals.

Rating : 0

Carrot

Carrots, naturally gluten-free, offer a wealth of nutrients, including beta carotene, fiber, and antioxidants. These vibrant root vegetables rank low on the glycemic index and are versatile in both raw and cooked forms. Their gluten rating is zero, making them a safe and nutritious choice for those adhering to a gluten-free diet. Carrots add crunch to salads, sweetness to soups, and serve as a wholesome snack.

Rating : 0

Cauliflower

Cauliflower, a versatile vegetable, ranks as a naturally gluten-free option. Its mild flavor and adaptable texture make it a favorite in gluten-conscious diets. Rich in fiber, vitamins, and antioxidants, cauliflower serves as a nutritious substitute for gluten-containing grains in recipes. From cauliflower rice to pizza crusts, its low gluten rating (zero gluten content) positions it as a valuable ingredient for those seeking gluten-free alternatives in their meals.

Rating : 0

Celery

Celery is naturally gluten-free, making it a safe choice for those with celiac disease or gluten sensitivity. This versatile vegetable contains no gluten, ensuring it won't trigger adverse reactions. Its crisp texture and mild, slightly peppery flavor make it a great addition to salads, soups, or as a crunchy snack. Whether raw or cooked, celery remains a nutritious and gluten-free option for various culinary uses.

Rating : 0

Cheese

Cheese, in its pure form, is naturally gluten-free. However, certain processed or flavored cheeses might contain additives that could potentially introduce gluten. Always check the label for any added ingredients or flavorings, as some cheese varieties, especially pre-packaged shredded or flavored options, might include additives with gluten. Opt for plain, unflavored cheese or those labeled explicitly as gluten-free to ensure they fit within a gluten-free diet.

Rating : 1

Cherry

Cherries are naturally gluten-free, holding no traces of the protein. This delicious fruit ranks as a safe option for those adhering to a gluten-free diet. Rich in antioxidants, fiber, and vitamins, cherries provide a sweet, tart flavor and versatile use in various dishes. Whether enjoyed fresh, dried, or as a juice, cherries stand as a gluten-free delight, contributing to a healthy and diverse diet without any gluten-related concerns.

Rating : 0

Chicken

Chicken, a versatile protein, is naturally gluten-free. However, caution is advised when purchasing pre-marinated or processed chicken products, as they might contain gluten-based ingredients in seasonings or coatings. Always check labels for any gluten-containing additives. Opting for fresh, unprocessed chicken or those explicitly labeled "gluten-free" ensures a safe choice for individuals adhering to a gluten-free diet.

Rating : 1

Chocolate

Chocolate, a beloved treat, varies in its gluten content based on its ingredients and manufacturing processes. Pure, unadulterated chocolate derived from cocoa beans is naturally gluten-free. However, cross-contamination can occur during processing, especially in products with added ingredients like flavorings or fillings. To ensure gluten-free chocolate, opt for brands that specifically label their products as "gluten-free" or look for certifications denoting adherence to gluten-free standards.

Rating : 2

Coconut

Coconut, a versatile and nutrient-rich fruit, ranks as a naturally gluten-free food. Both the flesh and milk derived from coconuts are inherently devoid of gluten, making them safe choices for those adhering to a gluten-free diet. Whether consumed raw, shredded, as coconut flour, or in the form of coconut oil or milk, coconut products remain excellent gluten-free options, allowing individuals with gluten sensitivities to enjoy their nutritional benefits worry-free.

Rating : 0

Cookie

Indulge in gluten-free cookies, crafted meticulously without wheat or its derivatives. These delightful treats embody flavors like almond flour chocolate chip or coconut macaroon, ensuring a delectable experience minus the gluten. Look for certifications like "Certified Gluten-Free" to guarantee a safe, enjoyable snack. Savor every bite of these cookies, free from gluten concerns, and relish the sweet pleasures of a delicious, worry-free treat.

Rating : 1

Corn

Corn is a naturally gluten-free grain, scoring a safe rating for those avoiding gluten. Its versatility makes it a staple in gluten-free diets. Used as flour, cornmeal, or whole kernels, it offers an excellent base for various dishes, from tortillas to polenta. However, be cautious with processed corn products, as cross-contamination can occur during manufacturing. Always choose certified gluten-free corn products to ensure they meet gluten safety standards.

Rating : 0

Croissant

Croissants are a classic pastry known for their flaky, buttery layers. However, they typically contain gluten due to the wheat flour used in their preparation. Unfortunately, this gluten content makes them unsuitable for those with celiac disease or gluten sensitivity. Gluten-free alternatives made with alternative flours like almond or tapioca aim to replicate the texture and taste, offering a similar experience without the gluten content.

Rating : 2

Cucumber

Cucumbers are naturally gluten-free, containing no measurable gluten levels. These crisp and refreshing veggies are excellent for gluten-sensitive individuals or those with celiac disease. Packed with hydration, vitamins, and antioxidants, cucumbers are a versatile addition to salads, sandwiches, or as a standalone snack. Their gluten-free status makes them a safe and nutritious choice for those adhering to a gluten-free diet without worrying about gluten contamination.

Rating : 0

Date

Dates are naturally gluten-free fruits, providing a sweet and nutritious option for those following a gluten-free diet. As whole, unprocessed fruits, dates don't contain gluten. They are a versatile ingredient, adding natural sweetness to recipes like energy bars, smoothies, and desserts. Always check for added ingredients or processing methods if purchasing processed or packaged date products to ensure they remain gluten-free.

Rating : 1

Donut

Donuts typically contain high levels of gluten due to their wheat flour base. The gluten content in traditional donuts poses a concern for individuals with gluten-related disorders. However, gluten-free versions made with alternative flours like rice, almond, or coconut flour provide a delicious option for those following a gluten-free diet. It's essential to check labels or inquire about ingredients to ensure the donuts meet specific gluten-free standards.

Rating : 3

Dragon Fruit

Dragon fruit, a vibrant tropical fruit, is naturally gluten-free. Its unique appearance with pink or yellow skin and speckled flesh contains tiny, edible seeds similar to those in kiwi. Rich in antioxidants, vitamins, and fiber, it's a nutritious choice. Regarding gluten, like most fruits, dragon fruit is inherently gluten-free, making it a safe option for those following a gluten-free diet, devoid of the protein that triggers reactions in sensitive individuals.

Rating : 0

Egg

Eggs are naturally gluten-free, containing no gluten proteins. They're a versatile and nutritious food, rich in protein, vitamins, and minerals. Whether scrambled, boiled, or used in baking, eggs pose no risk of gluten contamination. However, caution is needed with certain egg dishes or processed egg products that might contain added ingredients, so always check labels for any potential gluten-containing additives or cross-contamination risks.

Ratings : 1

Eggplant

Eggplant, a versatile and nutrient-rich vegetable, stands naturally gluten-free. High in fiber, vitamins, and antioxidants, it's a gluten-safe choice for various diets. This low-calorie veggie is a staple in Mediterranean cuisine, lending itself to dishes like eggplant parmesan or grilled eggplant salads. It's vital to note that in its unprocessed, unseasoned form, eggplant is inherently gluten-free, making it a fantastic addition to gluten-conscious meal plans.

Rating : 0

Fennel

Fennel, a flavorful herb with a mild licorice taste, is naturally gluten-free. This versatile plant, with its bulb, stalks, and fronds, rates as a safe option for those on a gluten-free diet. Rich in fiber, vitamins, and antioxidants, fennel adds depth to dishes without any gluten concerns. Whether used raw in salads, roasted with vegetables, or as a seasoning, fennel stands as a gluten-free culinary delight.

Rating : 0

Fig

Figs, known for their sweet taste and chewy texture, are naturally gluten-free. These nutrient-dense fruits contain vitamins, minerals, and dietary fiber, making them a wholesome addition to a gluten-free diet. Their low gluten rating ensures they're safe for individuals sensitive to gluten or with celiac disease. Figs can be enjoyed fresh or dried, adding a delightful sweetness to both sweet and savory dishes without the worry of gluten content.

Rating : 0

Garlic

Garlic, a versatile ingredient, is inherently gluten-free. Its rating on the gluten scale is zero, making it safe for those with celiac disease or gluten sensitivity. Packed with flavor and nutrients, garlic enhances various dishes without posing gluten-related risks. However, caution should be exercised with pre-prepared or processed garlic products, as additives or seasoning blends might introduce gluten. Always check labels to ensure purity for a gluten-free diet.

Rating : 0

Grape

Grapes, naturally gluten-free, are a sweet and juicy fruit. They're free from gluten and safe for those with celiac disease or gluten sensitivity. Rich in antioxidants, vitamins, and minerals, grapes are a nutritious snack or addition to salads, providing health benefits without any gluten-related concerns.

Rating : 0

Grapefruit

Grapefruit, a citrus powerhouse, stands gluten-free. Rich in vitamins, fiber, and antioxidants, it's a tangy delight often enjoyed fresh or juiced. Its zesty flavor boosts immunity and aids digestion. Naturally free from gluten, it's a safe choice for those with gluten sensitivities or celiac disease.

Rating : 0

Green Bean

Green beans are naturally gluten-free, scoring a perfect zero on the gluten scale. These crisp and nutritious veggies offer fiber, vitamins, and minerals without any gluten concerns. They're versatile in recipes, adding a crunch to salads or making a flavorful side dish, perfect for gluten-free diets.

Rating : 0

Guava

Guava, a tropical fruit, contains no gluten. This nutrient-packed delight offers vitamins C and A, fiber, and antioxidants. Its low glycemic index aids blood sugar control. Guavas come in various types, from sweet to tangy, making them versatile for snacks, desserts, or refreshing beverages.

Rating: 0.

Hamburger

A classic hamburger, consisting of a beef patty, lettuce, tomato, and onion, typically rates as gluten-free. However, it's crucial to note potential sources of gluten, such as the bun. Opt for a gluten-free bun or lettuce wrap to ensure the entire burger remains free from gluten-containing ingredients.

Rating : 1

Hazelnut

Hazelnuts are naturally gluten-free. They're nutrient-dense, packed with healthy fats, vitamins, and minerals. Hazelnuts rank low on the glycemic index, making them a favorable choice for those managing blood sugar levels. They're an excellent gluten-free ingredient for baking or enjoyed as a healthy snack.

Rating : 0

Honeydew

Honeydew, a refreshing fruit, is naturally gluten-free, making it a safe choice for those with gluten sensitivities. With its sweet, juicy flesh and high water content, this melon not only delights taste buds but also presents a low-risk option on the gluten-free rating scale, providing a delicious, worry-free snack.

Rating : 0

Ice Cream

Ice cream, a beloved treat, varies in gluten content. While basic flavors like chocolate or vanilla are often gluten-free, watch for additives or mix-ins like cookie dough or brownie pieces, which may contain gluten. Check labels or opt for certified gluten-free brands for a safer indulgence.

Rating : 2

Jalapeño

Jalapeños, those spicy green wonders, are naturally gluten-free. These fiery peppers add zest to dishes without containing gluten. Whether diced, pickled, or stuffed, jalapeños provide a flavor punch without any worries about gluten content, making them a safe and flavorful addition to gluten-free diets.

Rating : 0

Jackfruit

Jackfruit, a tropical fruit, is naturally gluten-free. Its versatile nature makes it a meat alternative in vegan cuisine due to its texture. It contains no gluten, making it suitable for those with celiac disease or gluten sensitivities, offering a flavorful, plant-based option for various dishes.

Rating : 0

Jicama

Jicama, a crisp root vegetable, is naturally gluten-free. With its mild, sweet taste and crunchy texture, jicama makes a versatile addition to gluten-free diets. Rich in fiber, vitamins, and minerals, it's an excellent choice for salads, slaws, or as a raw snack.

Rating : 0

Kale

Kale, a nutrient powerhouse, ranks naturally gluten-free. Rich in vitamins A, C, K, and minerals, it's a versatile leafy green suitable for various diets. With zero gluten, it's a valuable addition, offering antioxidants and fiber while complementing gluten-free meals, making it ideal for celiac-friendly dishes.

Rating : 0

Kaleidoscope Carrots (a variety of carrots)

Kaleidoscope Carrots, a vibrant heirloom variety, boast hues of purple, red, yellow, and orange. These naturally gluten-free root vegetables offer antioxidants, vitamins, and a sweet, earthy taste. Their diverse colors hint at a rich spectrum of nutrients, perfect for adding color and nutrition to gluten-free dishes.

Rating : 0

Kiwi

Kiwi, a nutrient powerhouse, is naturally gluten-free. This fuzzy fruit is a rich source of vitamin C, fiber, and antioxidants. Its low glycemic index makes it a great choice for a balanced diet, providing essential nutrients without containing any gluten, perfect for gluten-sensitive individuals.

Rating : 0

Lasagna

Lasagna, a classic Italian dish, traditionally contains gluten due to wheat-based pasta sheets. However, gluten-free lasagna utilizes alternatives like rice or corn noodles, ensuring a safe option for those with gluten sensitivities. Pairing with gluten-free sauces and fillings, it offers a delicious, celiac-friendly meal.

Rating : 2

Lemon

Lemons are naturally gluten-free, scoring a perfect zero on the gluten-rating scale. These citrus powerhouses provide vitamin C, antioxidants, and a tangy flavor to dishes and beverages. They're a versatile addition, enhancing flavors without any gluten concerns, making them ideal for gluten-free diets.

Rating : 0

Lettuce

Lettuce, a staple salad green, is inherently gluten-free. Its crisp, leafy texture makes it versatile for salads, wraps, and sandwiches. With zero gluten content, lettuce is a safe and refreshing option for those following a gluten-free diet, offering essential nutrients like vitamins A and K.

Rating : 0

Lychee

Lychee, a tropical fruit with a sweet, floral taste, is naturally gluten-free. It's a delicious source of vitamin C and antioxidants. Like most fruits, lychee doesn't contain gluten, making it a safe and enjoyable choice for those following a gluten-free diet or with gluten sensitivities.

Rating : 0

Macadamia Nut

Macadamia nuts are naturally gluten-free, making them a safe choice for those following a gluten-free diet. These creamy, buttery nuts offer a rich source of healthy fats, antioxidants, and minerals, serving as a versatile ingredient or a delightful snack without any gluten-related concerns.

Rating : 0

Mango

Mangoes, deliciously sweet and juicy, are naturally gluten-free. This tropical fruit is packed with vitamins A and C, fiber, and antioxidants. A perfect addition to salads, smoothies, or enjoyed on its own, mangoes contain no gluten, making them a safe and delightful choice for gluten-sensitive individuals.

Ratings : 0

Mushroom

Mushrooms, versatile and gluten-free, offer earthy flavors in various cuisines. Naturally lacking gluten, they're safe for those with celiac disease or gluten sensitivity. Rich in nutrients, mushrooms like portobellos and shiitakes elevate dishes without adding gluten, making them a fantastic choice for diverse, gluten-conscious diets.

Rating : 0

Nachos

Nachos, a popular Tex-Mex dish, typically feature gluten-free corn tortilla chips as the base. However, caution is needed with toppings like cheese, sauces, and seasoned meats, as they might contain gluten. Opt for certified gluten-free ingredients.

Rating : 1

Nectarine

Nectarines, a gluten-free fruit, boast a juicy, sweet taste akin to peaches. These nutrient-rich gems offer vitamins A and C, fiber, and antioxidants. Naturally free of gluten, they're a delicious addition to gluten-conscious diets, providing a flavorful and nutritious snacking or dessert option.

Rating : 0

Oatmeal

Oatmeal, a breakfast staple, is naturally gluten-free but can be contaminated during processing. Opt for certified gluten-free oats to ensure they haven't come into contact with gluten-containing grains. These oats are safe for most individuals with celiac disease or gluten sensitivity, offering a nutritious morning option.

Rating : 1

Olive

Olive, a versatile fruit prized for its oil and flavor, is naturally gluten-free. Its rating regarding gluten is zero, making it a safe choice for those with gluten sensitivities or celiac disease. Whether whole, pressed into oil, or used in various dishes, olives are a gluten-free delight.

Rating : 0

Olive Oil

Olive oil, a staple in many cuisines, is naturally gluten-free. Its extraction from olives ensures no gluten contamination. When purchasing, opt for reputable brands and check labels to confirm the absence of additives or cross-contamination risks, ensuring a safe gluten-free cooking or dressing option.

Rating : 0

Onion

Onions, a versatile kitchen staple, naturally lack gluten, making them a safe choice for gluten-free diets. These flavorful bulbs are packed with antioxidants and nutrients. Their low gluten rating ensures they're a fantastic addition to various dishes without triggering gluten-related issues for sensitive individuals.

Rating : 0

Orange

Oranges are naturally gluten-free, making them a safe choice for those following a gluten-free diet. They contain no gluten or gluten-containing ingredients. Enjoyed for their tangy sweetness and rich vitamin C content, oranges are a refreshing and healthy addition to any gluten-free meal plan.

Rating : 0

Pancake

Pancakes can vary in gluten content. Traditional recipes use wheat flour, high in gluten. Opt for gluten-free alternatives like rice or almond flour for a lower gluten rating. Check labels or recipes labeled "gluten-free" to savor fluffy pancakes without the gluten concerns.

Rating : 1

Papaya

Papaya is a tropical fruit packed with antioxidants, vitamins, and enzymes aiding digestion. Naturally gluten-free, it's safe for those with gluten sensitivities or celiac disease. With its low allergenic potential, it's a delightful addition to gluten-free diets, offering sweetness, fiber, and essential nutrients without gluten concerns.

Rating : 0

Pasta

Papaya, a tropical fruit, is naturally gluten-free. Rich in vitamins A, C, and antioxidants, it supports digestion and boosts immunity. Its low gluten rating (none detected) makes it a safe, nutritious choice for those following a gluten-free diet, offering a sweet and vibrant addition to meals.

Rating : 0

Peach

Peaches are naturally gluten-free, containing no gluten or gluten-related proteins. They're a delicious, juicy fruit rich in vitamins, fiber, and antioxidants. Enjoyed fresh or in various dishes, peaches make a healthy, celiac-safe option for those adhering to a gluten-free diet.

Rating : 0

Pear

Pears are naturally gluten-free, providing a sweet and juicy treat. With no gluten concerns, they're a safe choice for those on a gluten-free diet. Packed with fiber, vitamins, and antioxidants, pears offer a delicious and nutritious addition to meals, snacks, or desserts without any gluten worries.

Rating : 0

Peas

Peas, whether green, snow, or snap, are naturally gluten-free, making them safe for those with gluten intolerances. These versatile legumes pack fiber, protein, and essential nutrients. Their gluten rating is zero, offering a nutritious addition to soups, salads, or side dishes.

Rating : 0

Pepper

Pepper, whether black, white, or red, is inherently gluten-free. It's a versatile spice derived from peppercorns and doesn't contain gluten. Always check for potential cross-contamination or added gluten in spice blends or pre-ground pepper, ensuring they're certified gluten-free for sensitive individuals.

Rating : 0

Pineapple

Pineapple is a naturally gluten-free fruit known for its sweetness and tang. Rich in vitamin C, antioxidants, and enzymes, it's safe for a gluten-free diet. With no gluten content, pineapple is a versatile ingredient for both sweet and savory dishes, offering a tropical flavor boost without gluten concerns.

Rating : 0

Pizza

Pizza's gluten content varies. Traditional crust contains gluten from wheat flour, rating high on the gluten scale. However, gluten-free alternatives, made with rice, tapioca, or almond flour, offer low or no gluten. Check labels for "gluten-free" certification to enjoy pizza without gluten concerns, suiting various dietary needs.

Rating : 2

Plum

Plums are naturally gluten-free, offering a sweet and juicy treat packed with vitamins and antioxidants. Their low glycemic index and fiber content aid digestion. When fresh, dried, or in preserves, plums contain no gluten, making them a safe and delicious choice for those following a gluten-free diet.

Rating : 0

Popcorn

Popcorn is a naturally gluten-free whole grain, making it a safe and delicious snack for those with gluten sensitivities or celiac disease. Its rating is zero on the gluten scale, offering a guilt-free, crunchy treat. Ensure to choose plain or homemade varieties, as flavored versions may introduce gluten-containing additives.

Rating : 0

Potato

Potatoes are naturally gluten-free, making them a safe choice for those with gluten-related disorders. Rich in vitamins, minerals, and fiber, potatoes contribute to a balanced diet. From mashed potatoes to roasted wedges, they offer versatile gluten-free options, ensuring a flavorful and satisfying addition to gluten-free meals.

Rating : 0

Pomegranate

Pomegranate, a vibrant and nutrient-rich fruit, is naturally gluten-free. Bursting with antioxidants, it's a delicious addition to gluten-free diets. Its seeds are not only a flavorful snack but also add a delightful crunch to salads and desserts. Packed with health benefits, pomegranate is a gluten-free superfood enjoyed for its taste and nutritional value.

Rating : 0

Pumpkin

Pumpkin is naturally gluten-free, making it a versatile and nutritious choice for those with gluten sensitivities. Rich in vitamins, minerals, and fiber, pumpkin adds depth to both sweet and savory dishes. Its neutral gluten rating ensures a safe and flavorful addition to a gluten-free diet, offering culinary flexibility.

Rating : 0

Quinoa

Quinoa, a versatile gluten-free grain, stands out for its exceptional nutritional profile. Rich in protein, fiber, and various essential nutrients, quinoa is a powerhouse for those on a gluten-free diet. Its low gluten content, classified as gluten-free by international standards, makes it a staple for individuals with celiac disease or gluten sensitivity.

Rating : 0

Quince

Quince is a naturally gluten-free fruit with a unique flavor profile, resembling a blend of apples and pears. Rich in fiber, vitamins, and antioxidants, quince is a versatile ingredient for jams, jellies, and desserts. As a whole food, it naturally contains no gluten, making it a safe and delicious addition to gluten-free diets.

Rating : 0

Radish

Radishes are naturally gluten-free, making them an excellent choice for those following a gluten-free diet. Low in calories and high in fiber, radishes add a crisp, peppery flavor to salads and dishes. Their gluten rating is zero, ensuring they're safe for individuals with celiac disease or gluten sensitivity.

Rating : 0

Raisin

Raisins, derived from dried grapes, are inherently gluten-free. Their natural state poses no gluten concerns. However, when choosing flavored or coated varieties, it's crucial to check labels for potential gluten-containing additives. Always opt for products labeled "gluten-free" to ensure a safe choice for those with gluten sensitivities or celiac disease.

Rating : 1

Raspberry

Raspberries are naturally gluten-free, making them a safe and delicious option for those following a gluten-free diet. Bursting with antioxidants, fiber, and vitamins, these succulent berries are not only a flavorful addition to meals but also a nutritious choice for snacks and desserts, enhancing both taste and well-being.

Rating : 0

Rambutan

Rambutan, a tropical fruit native to Southeast Asia, is naturally gluten-free. With a sweet and juicy flavor, its translucent flesh surrounds a single seed.

Enjoyed fresh, this gluten-free delight provides a tasty and nutritious option for those with gluten sensitivities, contributing to a diverse and flavorful diet.

Rating : 0

Rice

Rice is a gluten-free staple, earning it a top rating in gluten awareness. This versatile grain, whether brown, white, or wild, serves as a crucial component in gluten-free diets. Rich in carbohydrates and a source of energy, rice is an excellent foundation for various dishes without triggering gluten-related issues for those with sensitivities.

Rating : 0

Sausage

Sausages, a popular meat product, may vary in gluten content. Always check labels for gluten-free indications. Opt for sausages with "gluten-free" labeling or those certified by recognized gluten-free organizations to ensure a safe choice for individuals with celiac disease or gluten sensitivity. Enjoy flavors without compromising dietary needs.

Rating : 2

Semolina

Semolina is a coarse flour typically made from durum wheat, boasting a high gluten content. It's commonly used in pasta, couscous, and some bread recipes. The gluten in semolina provides elasticity and structure, yielding products with a satisfying texture. However, it's unsuitable for those on a gluten-free diet due to its gluten-rich nature.

Rating : 3

Spinach

Spinach is a gluten-free powerhouse, providing a nutrient-dense option for those with gluten sensitivities. With a gluten rating of zero, it's a versatile leafy green that adds vitamins, minerals, and antioxidants to your diet. Enjoy spinach raw in salads, sautéed as a side, or blended into smoothies for a healthful boost.

Rating : 0

Squash

Squash, a versatile and nutritious vegetable, is inherently gluten-free. Whether it's butternut, acorn, or spaghetti squash, these varieties provide essential vitamins and antioxidants without any gluten content. Enjoyed roasted, pureed, or spiralized, squash offers a delicious and safe option for those following a gluten-free diet.

Rating : 0

Strawberry

Strawberries are naturally gluten-free, making them a safe choice for those with gluten sensitivities or celiac disease. Packed with vitamin C, antioxidants, and fiber, strawberries not only add a burst of sweetness to meals but also contribute to a nutritious and gluten-free diet.

Rating : 0

Taco

Tacos, a beloved dish, can be gluten-free when crafted with corn tortillas or certified gluten-free alternatives. Avoiding wheat-based tortillas is essential for those with gluten sensitivity. Incorporate gluten-free fillings like seasoned meats, fresh vegetables, and gluten-free sauces for a flavorful and safe taco experience.

Rating : 1

Tangerine

Tangerines are naturally gluten-free fruits, making them a safe and delicious option for those following a gluten-free diet. Rich in vitamin C, fiber, and antioxidants, tangerines offer a refreshing burst of citrus flavor without any gluten concerns. Enjoy this nutritious and gluten-free snack for a tasty and healthy treat.

Rating : 0

Tomato

Tomatoes are naturally gluten-free, containing no gluten or gluten-related proteins. These vibrant red fruits are rich in antioxidants, vitamins, and minerals. Whether enjoyed fresh in salads, as a base for sauces, or in various dishes, tomatoes are a versatile and healthy addition to a gluten-free diet.

Rating : 0

Tuna

Tuna, a nutritious source of protein and omega-3 fatty acids, is naturally gluten-free. Whether fresh or canned, tuna poses minimal risk of gluten contamination. However, caution should be exercised with flavored or processed tuna products, as additives and sauces may introduce gluten. Always check labels to ensure gluten-free status.

Rating : 1

Turkey

Turkey is a gluten-free protein source, making it suitable for individuals with celiac disease or gluten sensitivity. As a lean meat, it's rich in protein, vitamins, and minerals. Always ensure the preparation method avoids gluten-containing ingredients, ensuring a safe and nutritious option for those adhering to a gluten-free diet.

Rating : 0

Turnip

Turnips are naturally gluten-free, making them a safe and nutritious choice for those with gluten sensitivities. Packed with vitamins, minerals, and fiber, turnips add a crisp, slightly peppery flavor to various dishes. Whether roasted, mashed, or added to soups, turnips offer a gluten-free option for a delicious and wholesome culinary experience.

Rating : 0

Vanilla

Vanilla, extracted from orchids, is a gluten-free flavoring. Whether in the form of pure extract, paste, or whole vanilla beans, it adds a sweet and aromatic touch to both sweet and savory dishes. Be cautious with pre-packaged vanilla products, always checking labels for hidden gluten or cross-contamination risks.

Rating : 1

Waffle

Waffles, a delightful breakfast treat, can vary in their gluten content. Traditional waffles, made with wheat flour, are high in gluten. However, gluten-free alternatives using rice flour, almond flour, or other substitutes offer a delicious option for those with gluten sensitivities, ensuring a tasty morning indulgence without compromising dietary needs.

Rating : 2

Watermelon

Watermelon is a refreshing gluten-free choice. This juicy fruit, rated gluten-free, contains no traces of the protein. Packed with hydrating benefits, watermelon is not just a delicious summer treat;

it's a safe and enjoyable option for those with gluten sensitivities or celiac disease. Enjoy its sweetness worry-free!

Rating : 0

Yam

Yam is a versatile, gluten-free root vegetable with a low glycemic index. Packed with essential nutrients, it serves as an excellent source of complex carbohydrates, fiber, and vitamins. With its natural gluten-free status, yam provides a nutritious option for those adhering to gluten-free diets while offering a sweet and satisfying flavor.

Rating : 0

Yogurt

Yogurt is a versatile and nutritious gluten-free option, rich in probiotics for gut health. Ensure your yogurt is labeled "gluten-free" to avoid any potential contamination during processing. Read ingredient lists carefully, as flavored or mixed varieties may contain additives that need verification for gluten content.

Rating : 1

Zucchini

Zucchini, a versatile and gluten-free vegetable, is a nutritional powerhouse. Rich in vitamins A and C, potassium, and antioxidants, it adds a mild, crisp flavor to dishes. With a low gluten rating of zero, zucchini is an excellent choice for those adhering to a gluten-free diet, offering culinary flexibility and health benefits.

Ratings : 0

1. Education and Awareness: Educate yourself about sources of gluten and hidden ingredients. Learn to read food labels meticulously to spot gluten-containing elements or potential cross-contamination risks.

2. Whole Foods Emphasis: Focus on natural, unprocessed foods like fruits, vegetables, lean meats, fish, legumes, nuts, and gluten-free grains (quinoa, rice, corn) to ensure a well-rounded and nutritious diet.

3. Gluten-Free Alternatives: Explore and experiment with gluten-free versions of your favorite foods. Nowadays, there are numerous alternatives for pasta, bread, and baked goods made from gluten-free flours like almond, coconut, or chickpea.

4. Kitchen Safety: Maintain a gluten-free kitchen by using separate utensils, cookware, and cutting boards to prevent cross-contamination. Designate specific areas for gluten-free products to minimize accidental exposure.

5. Communicate Clearly: When dining out or attending social gatherings, communicate your

dietary needs clearly to chefs or hosts. Ask about ingredients and food preparation methods to ensure safety.

6. Plan Ahead: Plan meals and snacks in advance, especially when traveling or attending events. Bring along gluten-free snacks to avoid being caught without suitable options.

7. Support Networks: Connect with support groups or online communities where you can share experiences, recipes, and tips with others following a gluten-free lifestyle. It helps to have a network of understanding individuals who can provide advice or encouragement.

8. Stay Informed: Keep up with the latest information about gluten-free products, restaurants, and resources. Stay informed about any updates in labeling laws or gluten-free certifications.

CONCLUSION

The gluten-free food list provides a roadmap for individuals navigating dietary restrictions due to celiac disease or gluten sensitivity. This compilation of diverse, naturally gluten-free options empowers healthier choices, fostering a balanced and enjoyable culinary experience. From grains like quinoa to protein-rich meats and an array of fruits and vegetables, this list demonstrates that a gluten-free lifestyle need not compromise flavor or nutrition. The key lies in education, label awareness, and embracing the vast array of gluten-free alternatives available. By incorporating these foods into daily life, individuals can embark on a journey that not only supports their health needs but also opens doors to a world of delicious and satisfying gluten-free dining.

Please leave a positive rating and review on the amazon website after reading

Thank you

Sarah Thompson